Obesity and Self-Image

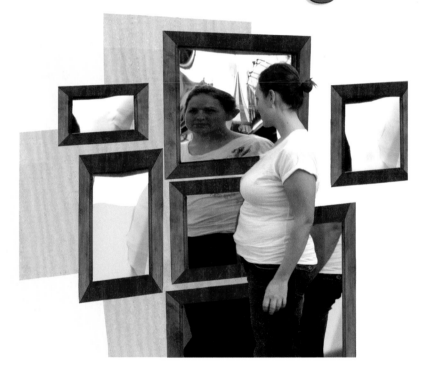

Judith Levin

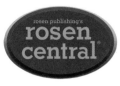

rosen publishing's
rosen central ®

New York

Published in 2009 by The Rosen Publishing Group, Inc.
29 East 21st Street, New York, NY 10010

Library of Congress Cataloging-in-Publication Data

Levin, Judith (Judith N.), 1956–
Obesity and self-image / Judith Levin.
    p. cm.—(Understanding obesity)
Includes bibliographical references and index.
ISBN-13: 978-1-4042-1768-3 (library binding)
1. Obesity—Psychological aspects. 2. Self-perception. I. Title.
RC552.O25.L478 2009
362.196'398—dc22

                             2007053005

Manufactured in the United States of America

Contents

Introduction

In 1890, an advertisement said, "Respectfully tell the ladies use 'Fat-Ten-U' food to get plump." This wonderful food supplement promised to make unhappy, thin women "Plump & Rosy with HONEST Fleshiness of Form." The ad includes the usual "before" and "after" pictures—except the "before" picture looks like a modern "after" picture. It is the thin woman who turns away in shame, and the plump woman who throws her head back in pride, showing off her beautiful fat body.

Those were the days! Imagine being told that thin people are the ones with a problem and that plumpness means you're strong, healthy, and beautiful. Men, too, were supposed to look solid and substantial.

This ad really is like the modern ones, though. It says: Don't look like you look now; look like this picture. It says you should be ashamed of how you look and also worry about your health. And it sells a product, which is made by a "professor," so it must be scientific. It promises magic, too: in just four weeks it will make you be a different shape and make you happy.

THE OBESITY CRISIS

In the beginning of the twenty-first century, people are not supposed to be obese. In 2005, the Centers for Disease Control and Prevention (CDC) estimated that about 112,000 people die each year from obesity-related illnesses. The number doesn't refer to children, but the article's authors did say that childhood and teen obesity will lead to life-shortening illnesses. The National Health and Nutrition Examination Survey says that about one out of three children and teens between the ages of two and nineteen are overweight or obese.

The CDC and many other organizations blame the obesity epidemic on fast foods, which are relatively inexpensive, available, and full of fat and sugar. They blame parents for not

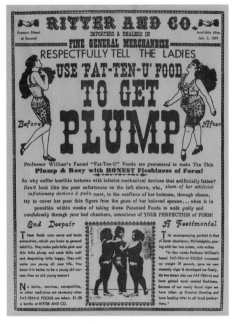

This ad from 1890 tells the woman on the left to eat "Fat-Ten-U" foods so that she doesn't have to be ashamed of her "poor thin figure."

being home to cook nutritious dinners. They also blame television and electronic games that encourage sedentary activity. Schools are blamed for not providing students with enough gym classes.

The United States has declared war on the "obesity epidemic." In 2007, the U.S. Congress debated bills, such as the Child Nutrition Promotion and School Lunch Protection Act, that would ban candy and sugary drinks from schools, but Congress has not passed the legislation yet. Some local school districts have regulated what is available to students in school cafeterias by offering healthy choices.

This "war" wouldn't be a bad thing if it really helped people to live healthier lives. Being overweight is associated with diseases

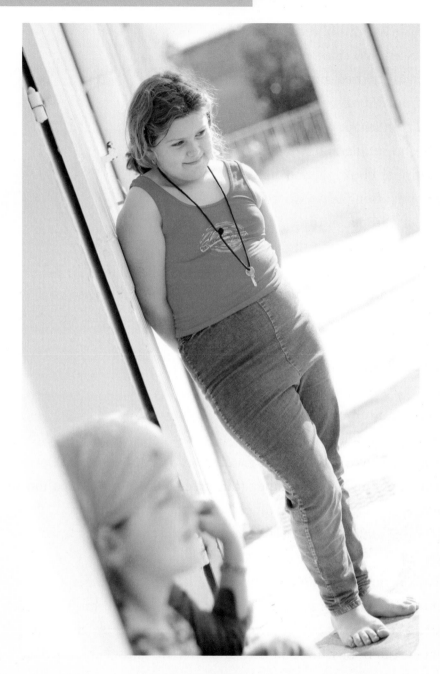

Years ago, parents and doctors might have said that this girl had "puppy fat" and would outgrow it. Now, they are more likely to worry about her health.

such as type 2 diabetes, high blood pressure, and high cholesterol. Of course no one wants these illnesses. Many young people are already worried about their weight. They look at pictures of celebrities and sports stars, and then they look at themselves. Maybe their parents are giving them a hard time about their eating, too. Perhaps their parents are giving them fast food for dinner or cooking food that might be very high in calories, and they are being teased about their weight at school.

Children and adults can get into big trouble at school or work if they harass someone for having a different skin color, being a different religion, or needing crutches. Young people tease and bully one another anyway, but inside they know that it's mean to tease someone who is in a wheelchair. After all, it's not his or her fault. What about people who weigh too much, though? Maybe it is their fault because they eat too much, don't exercise enough, or don't have self-control.

If you're the person being teased, maybe you even agree with them. Everybody knows it's better to be Harry Potter (skinny, kind, hardworking, and magic, even if he does have glasses and a scar) than his cousin Dudley (fat, greedy, lazy, stupid, and mean). Even Harry thinks that Dudley looks like a baby pig in his baby pictures and that it's *so funny* when a magician gives Dudley a pig's tail.

Of course you're not supposed to like Harry's mean cousin, but if Dudley was a black or Japanese stereotype instead of a fat stereotype, J. K. Rowling would have had to change how she wrote the books. Racism isn't allowed. Weightism is. After all, even the experts say it's wrong for you to be obese. They say "unhealthy," but that's still bad.

The years right before and during middle school have always been a tough time of life for young people and their bodies. It's the time your body changes, sometimes either too fast or too slowly. It's also a period of spending a whole lot of time looking at yourself in the mirror. Some kids skip meals to lose weight or go on "magic" diets that are supposed to melt the pounds away.

It is hard to maintain a good self-image when your body and mind are changing so fast. It's even harder if you have a weight problem, especially with the scary things the scientists and newspapers are saying. Is your weight making you sick? How should you look? Can you feel OK about yourself if you don't look that way? What should you do?

Chapter 1

Self-Image

Self-image is your mental picture of yourself. It's also how you think other people see you. A self-image isn't based just on how you look. (That's called body image.) Self-image is about *all* of who you are. Are you a leader or a follower? Are you mostly nice or kind of mean? Are you very intelligent or average or slow at schoolwork? In what ways are you brave and in what ways are you afraid? Do you like trying new things or are you more comfortable with the ones you already know?

Your self-image has been developing since you were a little child. It's not just how you feel on a great day or on a terrible, awful, no good, very bad day. It's your sense of your regular everyday you. Self-image does change over time and it can take a beating as you move toward your teens.

As you get older, you might be wondering what you are really like.

A mature and realistic self-image is something that people work on all their lives. What's more, you might be the only person who knows the truth about yourself. When you volunteer to help out at your little sister's birthday party, are you really doing it to please her and help out, or are you mostly thinking about how kind and helpful you are looking to others?

SELF-ESTEEM

Self-image is part of self-esteem. Self-esteem is how much you feel loved, valued, and accepted by other people. It's also about how much you value, love, and accept yourself. It can also be called self-respect or self-worth.

People with healthy self-esteem recognize and feel good about their strengths. They also recognize their weaknesses but can forgive themselves for not being perfect. If there's something they're not so good at, they'll try to figure out if they can do it better. (Stop teasing little brother so much? Maybe. Become a famous guitar player? Not if you've been taking lessons for two years and still can't tell if the thing's in tune.) They are willing to try new things and be bad at them for a while. This makes it more likely that they will learn to be better at them. Few people learn to ski without falling down or to cook without burning the bacon.

People with low self-esteem are likely to feel that they're not much good at things. Or maybe they are good at some things, but those aren't as important as what they are not good at. They focus on the negative and expect not to do very well. This can get in the way of their trying to do new things. They won't be any good. People will laugh. So why even try?

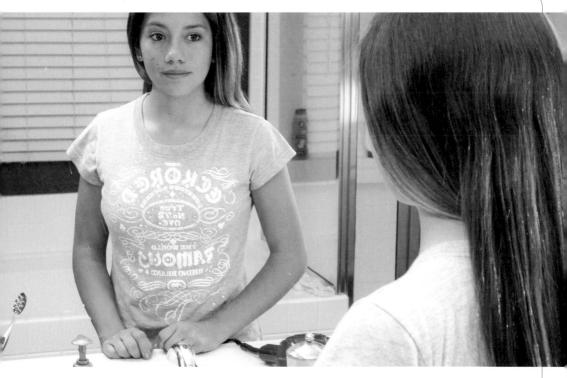

It's normal for teens to look at themselves in the mirror and wonder, How do I look? How do other people see me?

People with *exaggeratedly* high self-esteem also have an unrealistic sense of themselves. They may overvalue their strengths and feel they're doing really well even when they're not. This can make them annoying to other people. It's wonderful to feel good about yourself, but if you need to work harder at math or want to play a team sport, knowing your limitations is useful. It doesn't mean you feel bad about yourself; it means you need to work on your skills and maybe ask for help. Healthy self-esteem or self-regard is *realistic*. If you've got some strengths and some aspects about yourself that you'd like to improve, that's normal.

How Self-Image and Self-Esteem Develop

Self-image and self-esteem develop over time, partly in response to the messages people get from outside themselves. Children who grow up with parents who only tell them when they've done something wrong but never tell them when they've done well may grow up feeling that *nothing* they do is good enough. This can help create children (and adults) who seem to "have it all" but still feel terrible about themselves. It can be a surprise to find out that the attractive president of your class feels like a failure because no matter how much she does, it never seems to be enough to please her parents. A girl or boy like that may take in or "internalize" the voice that says that he or she is bad or a failure. He or she might achieve a lot or might give up trying to do anything. Some are able to turn off the voices that say they aren't good enough and to take pleasure in their achievements.

As people are growing up, they compare themselves to the people they see around them. They create an image of who they want to be and of which traits are worth having.

Body Image

Obviously, people of all shapes and sizes have been exposed to messages about how they should look, and looks are part of self-image. In teens, body image (how you look and how you think you look) is a big part of self-image. Weight is one of the ways that people are expected to look "right" or look like people on television look.

So do overweight young people always have poor self-esteem? No, but many worry about their bodies and feel bad about them.

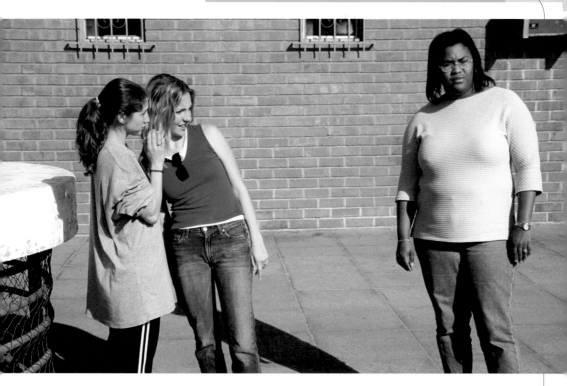

Overweight teens may find themselves excluded from some social groups as if their weight were a contagious illness.

Teens who have been teased for being obese are likely to feel bad about themselves, according to a research study published in the *Journal of Pediatrics and Adolescent Medicine.* Girls tend to worry more about being overweight than boys. One study by Daniel Kirschenbaum showed that perception of being overweight affected self-esteem. That means that young people who felt fat felt bad about themselves, even if they weren't really overweight. It's an easy time to feel fat. Watching television or reading magazines or looking at billboards, you see pictures of very skinny women and toned, bulked-up guys.

How Are People Supposed to Look?

Weight is just one part of their looks that people learn to worry about. In her book *The Beauty Junkies*, Alex Kuczynski writes about the growth of the cosmetic surgery business. The field of plastic surgery got its start after the Civil War (1861–1865), as doctors tried to help soldiers who had been injured in the conflict. Back then, a nose job meant that the doctor tried to make a new nose for someone who had his own shot off. Now, people—young and old, women and men—can have their noses done just to get one that looks "right." Also, they can change their teeth, ears, cheekbones, chins, toes, bottoms, tops, and belly buttons. They can pay to have their fat sucked away (liposuction) and, sometimes, injected in body parts that they think are too thin, like their lips. People can choose to have the smile of their favorite celebrity, instead of the smile of their dads. Kuczynski describes a party at which men had trouble finding their wives because all of the women there had the same hair, nose, lips, eyes, and clothes. It's not just young people who feel the pressure to look like everyone else.

"AM I FAT?"

The way many doctors and organizations define "overweight" and "obese" is according to something called the body mass index, or BMI. This is a number based on the relationship of people's height to their weight.

For people under the age of twenty, BMIs are also computed according to age and gender. Children and teens are still growing, and a healthy weight can be very different depending on someone's age and on whether he or she has just grown a lot or is about to. A young person who plays a lot of sports may weigh more because he or she has extra muscle, not extra fat.

If you use the metric system, your BMI is your weight (in kilograms) divided by the square of your height (in meters). In inches and pounds, you have to take your weight in pounds and divide by your height (in inches) squared, then multiply that number by 703. There are online calculators that will help you figure this out and tell you what the result means, but the result isn't really all the information you need. (One calculator can be found at: http://apps.nccd.cdc.gov/dnpabmi/calculator.aspx.)

The BMI (body mass index) calculator can be used to determine if a person is underweight, average, or overweight, but for young people, who are still growing, age and gender are also part of the calculation.

If your BMI has remained steady since you were a little kid, even if you're on the big side, it may be that you're just big. Bodies are *not* supposed to be all the same. If your BMI goes up every year or all of a sudden, though, then it's time to find out what is causing this change. (If someone's BMI drops very suddenly, then it's also time to find out what's causing the

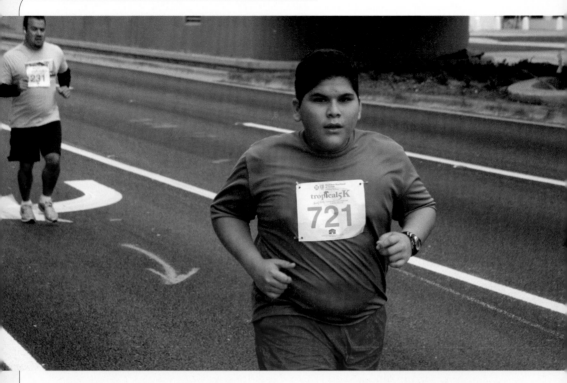

This teen is running a half marathon of 13.1 miles (21.1 kilometers). Only a doctor's exam could tell for sure, but if he eats well, he may be healthier than a thinner teen who sits in front of a computer all day.

change. Sudden weight loss can be caused by diabetes or by an eating disorder.) That doesn't just mean that as you get taller, you weigh more, but that you've gotten much heavier in relationship to your height.

Two groups of children and teens should be concerned about their weight for health reasons, according to the medical journal *Pediatrics*:

1. Young people who are heavier than ninety-five out of one hundred children who are their age and sex. This

is called the 95th percentile. They are considered overweight. The term "obese" is sometimes used.

2. Children who are heavier than 85–94 percent of kids who are their age and sex are considered "at risk for overweight." If young people are in this percentile and also have medical problems that may be related to weight, then they should make changes in their eating and activity that make them healthier. One medical problem is high blood sugar. This condition would suggest that they might develop type 2 diabetes or metabolic syndrome. (Metabolic syndrome is a collection of dangerous heart attack risk factors in a person, which include diabetes, abdominal obesity, high cholesterol, and high blood pressure.) Another possible problem is when being overweight makes it difficult to play sports or to walk for a half hour without getting out of breath.

Some people, including Paul Campos, author of *The Obesity Myth*, argue that doctors, schools, and parents should focus on *everyone* who is out of shape and doesn't eat a balanced diet, no matter what they weigh.

Chapter 2

Media Messages

It might be helpful to understand why the ladies in the "Fat-Ten-U" food ad were encouraged to be fat and why (and how) you are now taught to admire being skinny.

WHEN FAT WAS IN FASHION

In the past, the ability to store fatty tissue in the body easily helped people survive. For much of human history, food has been hard to produce, hard to store, and hard to move from place to place. Most people did more physical work than people do today, planting and harvesting crops by hand. There were few laborsaving machines. Also, people in climates with cold winters burned calories just trying to stay warm.

In many places, people didn't have much fat in their diets. Ordinary people (ones who weren't rich) ate less meat. It was expensive and hard to store. If they hunted or ate their farm animals, most of the animals were lean because they had had active lives, too.

So, in the past, it was easier to be thin than to be overweight or obese. Being overweight showed that you could afford to eat more calories than you burned. It was a sign of success and wealth. The painter Peter Paul Rubens (1577–1640) was so famous for his pictures of beautiful, billowy, fleshy ladies that "Rubenesque" is still a polite word for a plump or rounded woman. Paintings of the time sometimes show men with big stomachs, too.

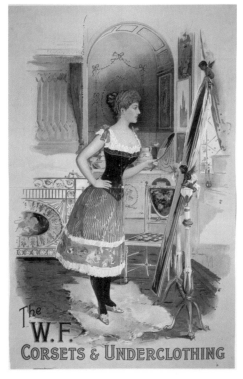

The fashion-conscious woman of the 1890s crushed her waist and ribs with a tightly laced corset. It was a dangerous fashion: the garment prevented the woman from breathing normally, since her lungs could not expand.

The "fat" ladies of the 1890 ad were supposed to be plump and rosy, but they were also supposed to have small waists and wore corsets that smashed in their stomachs. Some women even had surgery to have their lower ribs removed so that they would have perfect "hourglass" figures: big on the top and bottom, with a tiny waist. Their big tops and bottoms showed that their husbands (or fathers) could afford to buy expensive food and that they did not have to work hard. Their slender middles made

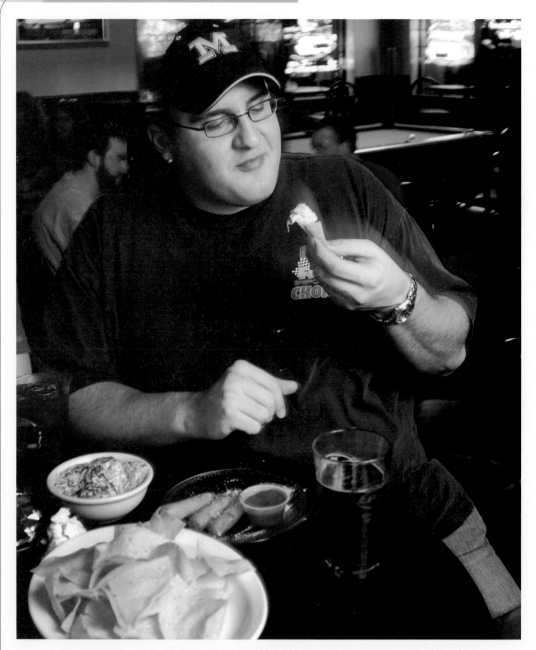

Modern high-fat, high-carbohydrate fast foods make it easy to gain weight. Very salty or sweet foods encourage people to eat long after they are full, especially if a salty food is paired with a sweet drink.

them look elegant and controlled. A nineteenth-century middle-aged businessman was supposed to be hefty and solid and look as though he ate a lot of beef. That showed that he was successful and healthy.

Why Thin Is In

It's harder to stay thin today, just as plumpness was harder for most people to achieve in the past. Now with all the high-calorie, high-fat, and high-carbohydrate foods available, it's easy for most people to put on weight. And it's cheaper foods that have more calories. Poorer people are more likely to be heavy than richer ones. Just as people once showed off their success by weighing more, they now show it off by weighing less (and less and less). Except for some people who easily burn off everything they can eat, weighing less shows that you have excellent self-control, perhaps work out at the gym, and eat relatively expensive foods—lean meats and fresh vegetables, for instance.

There's more pressure now to be thin than there was in the past to be overweight. It's easier to make something fashionable now. A hundred years ago, people might have seen fashion magazines a few times each year. Men and women who were servants or worked in shops saw what their employers and customers looked like. They could read about health and beauty, but they couldn't even see photographs because there was no way to print photos in a magazine or book. (Someone could draw a copy of the photo and print that.) Most working people didn't expect to look like rich ones. Now you're surrounded with images of skinny, muscular people, and the front pages of many weekly newspapers and magazines are dedicated to showing you which actress just gained two pounds.

How Ideal Body Images Get Distorted

The possibilities for conforming to a certain look are greater than they were, as the author of *The Beauty Junkies* shows. Young women can compare themselves with actresses and society women who have been made over by plastic surgery, trainers, and restrictive diets. Young men can compare themselves to actors who

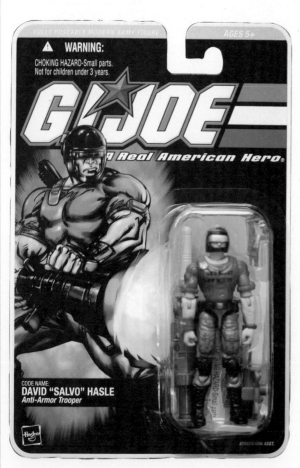

work out with trainers for hours each day or athletes who take steroids. Even the GI Joe toy has changed over the years, according to a study of action toys published in the *International Journal of Eating Disorders*. By 1998, the toy's muscles had grown so much that if you made him life-sized, he would have larger biceps than any bodybuilder in history.

Action figures for boys, such as G.I. Joe dolls, present them with an ideal body image that is as distorted as the one girls see in their Barbie dolls.

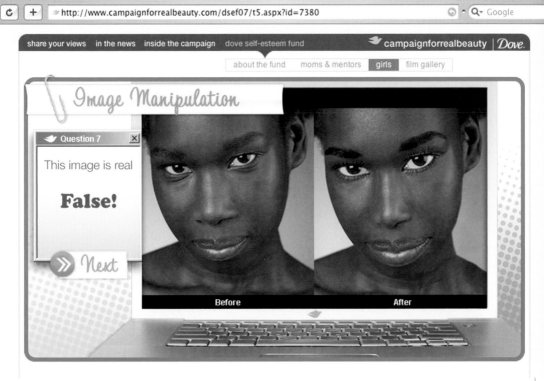

share your views   in the news   inside the campaign   dove self-esteem fund   campaignforrealbeauty | Dove.

about the fund   moms & mentors   girls   film gallery

Image Manipulation

Question 7

This image is real

False!

Next

Before | After

Dove's "campaign for real beauty" (www.campaignforrealbeauty.com) demonstrates how makeup and digital distortion create false ideals of how people should look. Even cosmetic surgery will not make a woman's eyes bigger.

It's also easier to misrepresent—to lie about—what people really look like. Dove's "real beauty" campaign offers online films that show how people's perceptions get so distorted about beauty. One of them shows, in fast motion, an ordinary-looking woman being turned into a glamorous advertisement. She is made up by a professional and has her hair changed and shaped and glued into place. After her picture is taken, the image is not only airbrushed to remove the pores on her skin but digitally altered to give her higher cheekbones and a longer neck. The film ends with the ad that shows a "beautiful" model who doesn't resemble the woman at all.

MIXED MESSAGES

The media bombard you with images of people you can't look like. At the same time, the media bombard you with ads for soft drinks, fast food, and sugary cereals. The food ads are as unrealistic as the "you-should-look-like-this" ads.

People who photograph food are called food stylists. Some of what they do can't be helped: the lights used in professional photography are hot, and foods dry out or melt. Still, an article in *Choice* (an Australian magazine similar to *Consumer Reports*) and a Web page from PBS might make you think twice about what's been done to make the food in an ad look good. Tricks include coating meat, fish, and vegetables with liquid soap or vegetable oil to make them glisten, spraying fabric protector on pancakes so the syrup doesn't soak in (or using motor oil instead of syrup), and placing cereal in white glue instead of milk so it won't get soggy.

The people who make advertisements also teach you to connect products with good feelings. The ads say (or show) that you should eat the product and then you'll be happy. You'll have friends. There's a toy in the box. Everyone smiles when they eat this. If your mom heats this in the microwave for you, it shows that she loves you. It's buttery/sugary/deliciously magic and the whole world will burst into song all around you if you eat it. (Well, that's what happens on television.) Also, you won't be overweight or obese, because the people eating the stuff on television are thin.

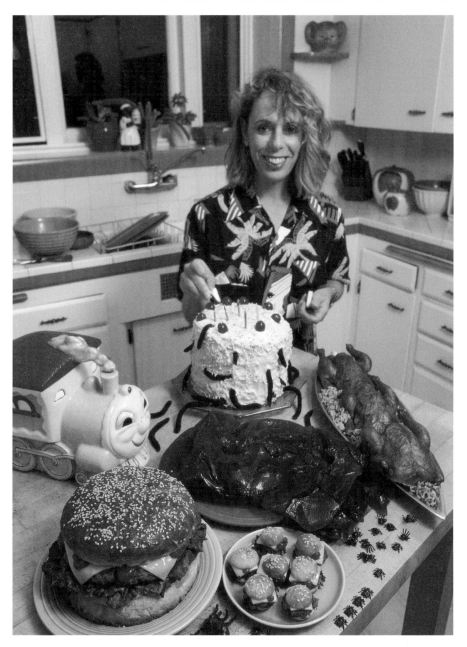

Food stylists create foods that photograph well and won't melt or dry out under hot studio lights. Sometimes, they also make foods look more delicious and tempting than they are in real life.

Myths and Facts

Myth: "You can't be too rich or too thin."

Fact: This famous saying is usually attributed to Wallis Simpson, Duchess of Windsor (1896–1986). She was an American divorcée who married the man who would have been King Edward VIII of England but who gave up the throne to marry her. She also said, "All my friends know I'd rather shop than eat." So, of course she preferred to be thin and rich. For everyone else, there really is such a thing as being "too thin." You could be too thin because of an eating disorder or too thin because you are struggling to keep a weight that is wrong for your body. You're supposed to have flesh. You're supposed to have muscle.

Myth: "No pain, no gain," as the old saying goes.

Fact: There are times when new habits aren't comfortable. If you decide to take better care of yourself, you will probably have to really think about what you're eating or how you're spending your time. It shouldn't hurt, though. If you're *painfully* hungry between meals, then you're not eating enough. If you're pushing yourself in the gym or running so hard that you have an ache that doesn't go away soon, then you're working out too hard. Make changes gradually. Make changes that you can live with comfortably.

Myth: You will be happy when you're thin.

Fact: Geneen Roth, who works with people on body image and eating issues, asked people in a workshop how many of them had lost weight and had been thin. Lots of them had. How many of them had felt fabulous when they'd lost weight? Only a few. How many of them believed that the next time they lost weight, they'd feel wonderful? Absolutely everyone. This, she suggests, is not a good idea. If you often think, "If only I were thinner," then you may have an unrealistic view of how losing weight will change your life. You may never be as thin as you'd like. You may never be thin at all. Your happiness can't depend on what the scale says.

In a recent study, Lisa Powell and other researchers studied the ads for food that children and teens see on television. For the two- to eleven-year-olds, 97.8 percent of the foods were high in fat, sugar, or salt. The ads that teens saw were only slightly better. How well do young people learn to pay attention to these messages? Very well. In August 2006, the television program *Dateline* discussed the question of whether food companies had any responsibility for the rise in obesity in the United States. In 2002, two teenaged girls sued McDonald's for making them fat. Many of the consumers interviewed on *Dateline* argued, as McDonald's had, that people make their own choices about what they eat. Law professor John Banzhaf and psychologist Susan Linn discussed how people's choices are influenced by advertising campaigns. Children learned to make unhealthy decisions based on advertising. *Dateline* filmed an experiment that looked at how three- and four-years-olds made decisions about what to eat. Almost all the children ate whatever the familiar cartoon characters told them to eat. They asked for a banana instead of a cupcake if the cartoon characters told them to. They also chose a rock for breakfast instead of the banana when the rock was decorated with cartoon character stickers.

So there are two sets of messages coming from the media:

1. You have to look like THIS—but "this" is not a way that most people are ever going to look. It's not even the way the real models look.
2. You really have to taste this doughnut and this burger and some fries and chocolate cereal with marshmallows in it for breakfast and a twenty-ounce soft drink with

a free refill, and the newest "coffee" drink that has six hundred calories in it but no coffee.

The teens who sued McDonald's lost. They couldn't prove that McDonald's had made them fat. But the *Dateline* episode concluded that companies really do influence people's eating choices in unhealthy ways. At the same time, you are told that your eating decisions are up to you. You should have self-control. You should make good choices.

For the sake of your self-image, your self-esteem, and your health, you have to be able to see through those mixed messages and figure out how to make choices that really are your own.

Chapter 3

The Experts on Obesity

The experts don't agree about how big a problem being overweight is or on what the solutions are. *The Journal of the American Medical Association* claimed in 2005 that there are 365,000 deaths each year related to poor diet and physical inactivity (the CDC has since revised that estimate to 112,000 obesity-related deaths per year). That larger number is repeated constantly by writers of books and magazine articles. In 2005, in the *New England Journal of Medicine*, S. Jay Olshansky and his colleagues published a study that said that obesity would cause the average life expectancy of Americans to fall. For the first time in two hundred years, children couldn't be expected to have a life span as long as that of their parents. The average life span could be as much as five years shorter. Many people use these numbers as evidence that a lot of people should go on a diet.

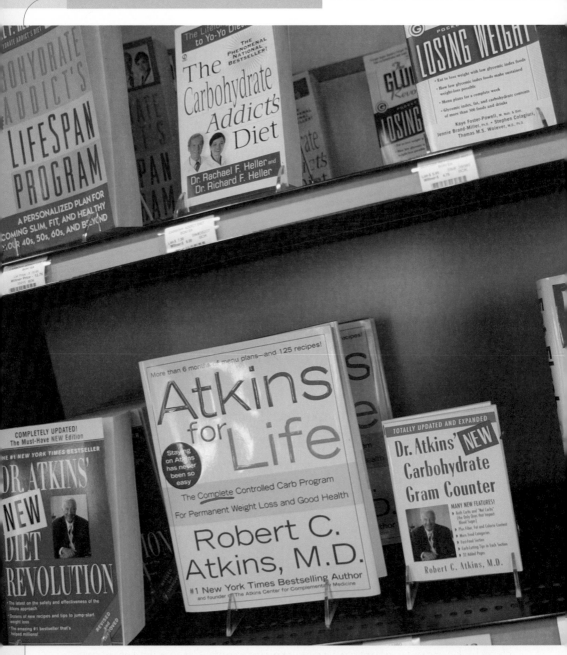

Every year, new diet books are published, based on current theories of how to lose weight. Many of the diets work, but as soon as people stop dieting, they regain the weight they have lost. Then they might buy another diet book.

Yet other experts say that the number is all wrong. Some argue that just as the food companies want to sell us their products, the obesity experts want to sell things, too. Sometimes, individuals are selling a diet book or product. In 2004, according to Marketdata Enterprises, Americans spent about $46 billion trying to lose weight. Others with an interest in obesity belong to respected organizations that receive money (much of it from people in the weight-loss industry) to do research on health problems.

Is Obesity an "Overblown Epidemic"?

In his 2005 *Scientific American* article "Obesity: An Overblown Epidemic?," W. Wayt Gibbs looked at a number of recent books that question whether obesity is as dangerous as many authorities are saying it is. For instance, in 2003, Dr. Julie Gerberding, director of the Centers for Disease Control and Prevention, claimed that obesity was a bigger problem than any epidemic in history, including the Black Plague in the Middle Ages and flu epidemics.

In *The Obesity Myth*, Paul Campos says the American Medical Association's estimated 300,000 deaths per year includes people who die because constant dieting has made their weight yo-yo up and down, which puts strain on the heart. It includes people who died because of diet drugs. He (and many others) have pointed to the evidence that most people who have been on "diets" lose weight only to gain it back—and more. "Is people's weight the real problem?" he asks. Campos argues that we should be paying attention to more than fat. This includes eating too much or eating non-nutritious food, not getting enough exercise, and lack of good health care.

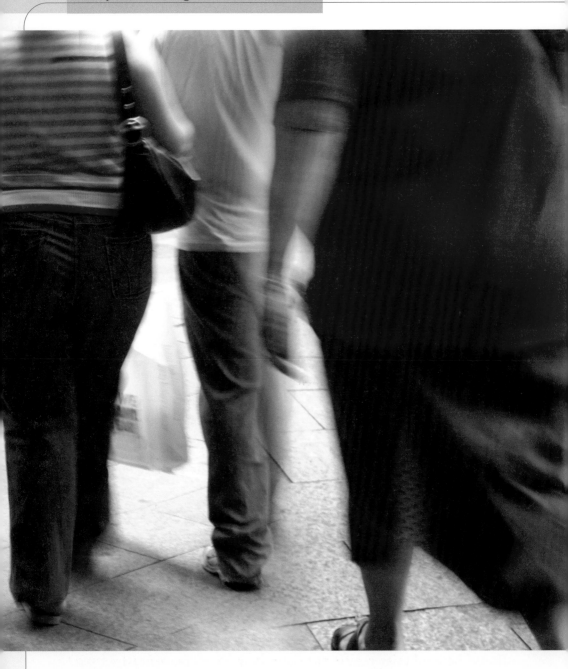

Americans are getting heavier, but should they worry about what the scale says or just make sure they are eating nutritious food and getting enough exercise? Experts disagree.

That might sound like different ways of saying the same thing: you have to eat right and you have to get exercise. There's a difference, though: Campos and others are saying that for good health you have to live a healthy lifestyle. That lifestyle may or may not lead you into the weight range that the body mass index recommends. He says that calling obesity a disease and telling people to lose weight creates huge numbers of people who are "sick" but can never get well because no one has figured out a way for most people to lose a lot of weight and keep it off. That's good for the people making money from dieters, but not good for the people's bodies or for their feelings about themselves. Different bodies are meant to be different weights.

Campos argues that obesity itself is not a disease. When the United States Department of Health and Human Services and the U.S. Department of Agriculture created a guide to nutrition, they wrote that excess body fat "leads to" at least ten diseases that can cause people to die earlier than they otherwise would have. "Leads to" means it *causes* these diseases. Instead, Campos argues, being overweight—especially very overweight—is *associated* with these diseases. He discusses scientific studies that show that often a very small weight loss makes people much healthier when they become active and eat wholesome foods.

What Scientific Studies (and Disagreements) Mean for You

If the rising obesity rate is not "a massive tsunami headed toward the United States," as David Lewis, one of the authors of a *New England Journal of Medicine* article about obesity has claimed, what does that mean for you?

Well, it is not an invitation to live on fast food until you're thirty or to get so little exercise that a flight of stairs poses a major challenge. Campos and others agree that Americans are getting heavier. Many—of all weights—could be healthier. Campos and Gibbs do raise the possibility that people (and their doctors and parents and classmates) have to be realistic about what a healthy weight is for each individual.

Chapter 4

Self-Image and Lifestyle Changes

Depending on what you are trying to do regarding your weight, you might need to consult with a doctor, nutritionist, or other adult.

Perhaps you know for a fact that you are eating more than you need to of foods that are high in calories but low in good nutrition. That is not an easy change to make, but if you want to drink less soda, eat more fruits and vegetables, and see what happens, that doesn't require a doctor's advice. Especially if you have gained weight and don't know why, then talking to a doctor is a good idea. A variety of medical conditions can cause someone to gain weight. In addition, a doctor can test your blood sugar, blood pressure, and cholesterol. A doctor can also tell you if there is any reason that you should be careful as you begin to be more active.

Another good resource for you is a nutritionist or another adult

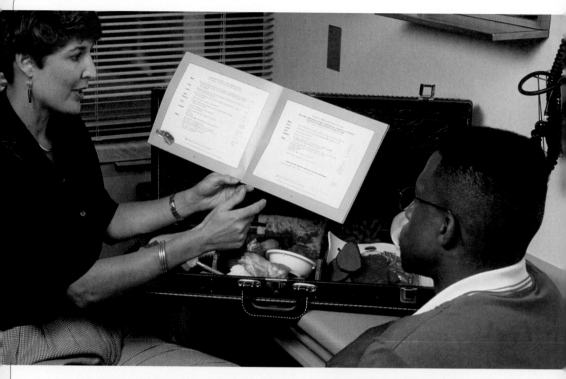

Nutritionists can help people improve their eating habits. They can also counsel people who want to limit their calories (while still eating nutritious foods) or who must eliminate foods to which they are allergic.

who knows about good eating habits. Nearly everyone thinks about eating fewer calories to lose weight, but food is the fuel that your body needs to function. Diets that cut out all carbohydrates or all fat (or tell you that you can have all the cabbage soup you want but nothing else) don't create good eating habits or give you all the nutrients you need to be healthy.

HOW NOT TO GO ON A DIET

Whatever plan you make for yourself cannot include denying yourself foods that you love, every day, forever, unless you have a medical condition that makes some foods genuinely dangerous to you. Otherwise, you are going to feel like the oldest failed dieters you've ever heard of: Adam and Eve just had to eat that apple, just because they were told they couldn't. "Forbidden fruit"—or ice cream—is going to torture you. The feeling of depriving yourself can easily lead to bingeing. If you know you can have an ice cream cone (or whatever you like best) sometimes, then you are less likely to eat a gallon of it in the middle of the night. Diets make people think about what they can't have. You need a plan you can live with.

MAKING A COMMITMENT

The decision to change your eating and exercise habits is a big commitment. Lots of people can starve themselves into weight loss, but few can maintain it. Anne Fletcher wrote *Weight Loss Confidential*, a book about how more than a hundred teens lost weight and kept it off. One of the teenagers was her son. Even though she is a dietician and filled the house with good-tasting, healthy foods and good advice, none of that made any difference until her son was ready to make a change. He and the other teens she spoke with told her the same thing: the interest in changing what they ate and how they lived had to come from them. No permanent change could come because their parents or their doctor told them to change. They had to be motivated.

What all of them did was get control over what they were eating and how they were living. Some of the teens spoke of "dieting" but all of them understood that they were making a permanent change in their lives. They weren't going on a diet for

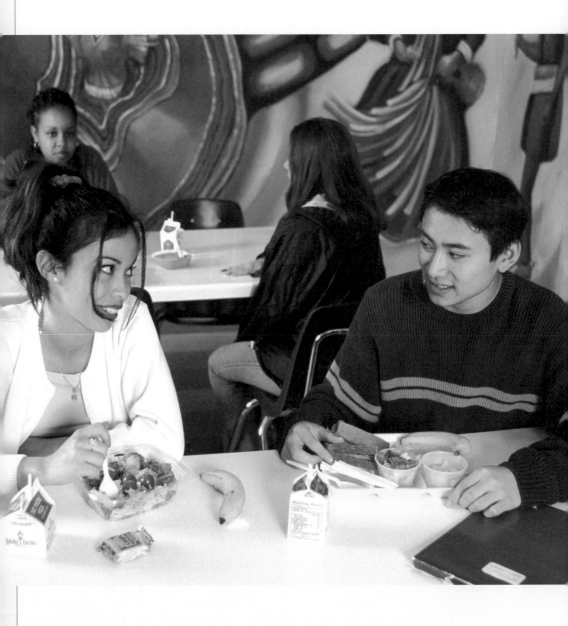

Teens cannot be forced to change their eating habits, but some schools are trying to help students make healthy choices.

a few weeks or even a few months. Many had already lost and regained the same pounds (and more) over and over again.

THE DANGERS OF A POOR SELF-IMAGE

A negative self-image and low self-esteem are likely to get in your way whether you're trying to lose weight or just eating better and moving more. They might make you too quick to say "I can't do it." Low self-esteem makes people critical of themselves, so it may make it harder for you to forgive yourself the day you absolutely lose it and eat everything you've promised yourself not to eat.

A negative self-image also makes it more likely that you'll focus on your problems and not pay attention to the good stuff about you. You might hate your fat thighs, but can you also love your shiny hair, not to mention your great taste in music and old movies? Not liking yourself is also going to make it harder to set realistic goals. "Perfect" isn't possible. No one can be that. You can't imagine that you will be a completely different person when you're thin or a completely different person when you've got better muscles.

What else is part of your self-image? Are you nice, or at least reasonably decent, to others? Are you good at something—a sport, a subject in school, an art such as painting or dancing? What are you like (not just your body, *you*)? Are you funny? Clever? Thoughtful? If your best friend was (or is) a person who is blind or you have a pen pal or talk to kids in an online chat room, how do those people "see" you?

What you can try to do is treat yourself, even your heaviest self, with kindness. Getting exercise and eating in a way that

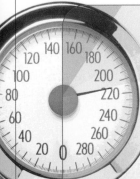

Ten Great Questions to Ask a Doctor or Nutritionist

1. What can I do if my parents are too critical of me when I'm already trying to change?

2. What can I do if my family is making it hard for me to change my habits because I know I have to eat differently from how we eat at home?

3. What can I do when I want to eat but I know I'm not really hungry?

4. Which of my eating habits can I change to be healthier?

5. What should I do about kids who tease me?

6. What can I do to stop thinking negative thoughts about myself and my body?

7. Are there local programs where people my age and weight can exercise comfortably, without people looking at us funny?

8. How can I work on making others more accepting of the fact that people are not all meant to be the same size and shape?

9. Do I need the support of a group, or can I change my habits by myself?

10. How do I know if I'm just feeling bad about myself because of my weight or because I'm depressed?

makes you healthy aren't to punish yourself. You're not starving yourself because you're obese/bad. You are taking better care of yourself, as you would take care of a good friend or your old dog. You do *not* need the "electronic conscience" that Hillel Schwartz describes in his book, *Never Satisfied*, about the history of diets and attitudes toward fat. Whenever you open the refrigerator door, he writes, it sneers, "Are you eating again? Shame on you! No wonder you look the way you do! Ha! Ha! Ha! You'll be sorry, fatty. Do yourself a favor: *shut the door*!"

If you've been struggling with your weight, you may already have a voice like that in your head. It may make you so unhappy and ashamed that you eat faster to drown it out.

IMPROVING YOUR SELF-IMAGE

Geneen Roth works with people on eating and body image. Many of the people in her workshops have been on diets for years. Some have struggled with eating disorders. She doesn't teach people to diet.

Roth became interested in people's feelings about their bodies and about food because of her own experiences with her weight and her negative self-image. In her article "Make Peace with Your Body," she says that she felt fat at 180 pounds (82 kilograms) and fat at 80 pounds (36 kg). She never felt that she looked good. Like many people who try and try to diet, Roth ended up not trusting herself or her food. She felt guilty whenever she ate foods that weren't on her diet, so she ate them secretly and in huge quantities. Bingeing just made her feel worse about herself.

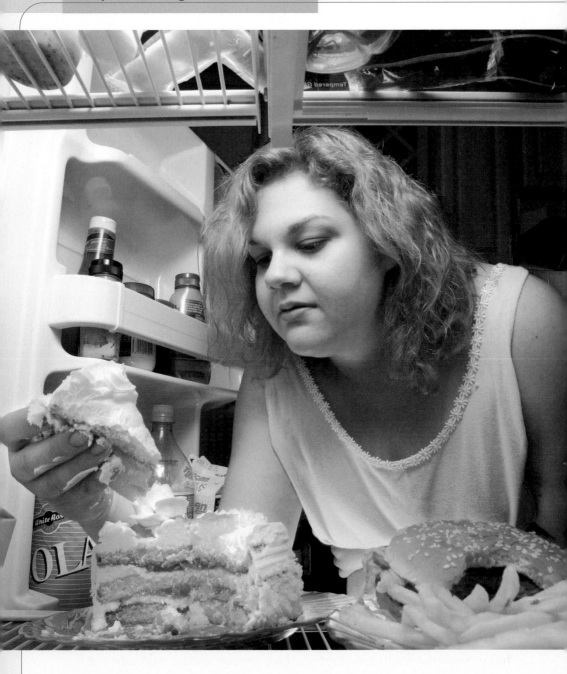

People who struggle with their weight may eat too much yet enjoy their food too little. Feeling guilty may cause them to eat more or even to binge.

EATING FOR HUNGER, EATING FOR COMFORT

Roth says people can relearn the difference between mouth hunger and stomach hunger: if your stomach is hungry, then you eat something. (Keeping in mind that it takes some time for a full stomach to signal your brain that it's full, so if you eat really fast, you're probably eating more than you're hungry for.) Roth calls the other "mouth hunger." Others call this emotional eating. It's when you eat because you're bored or blue or angry or tired.

It's not strange that you do this. You can often comfort a crying baby by putting a pacifier in his or her mouth. If the baby is truly hungry, then he or she will soon cry again, realizing he or she is not being fed. Otherwise, sucking on a pacifier or on a thumb is one of the first ways children learn to comfort themselves. Older children or adults may chew on their hair or bite a pencil or their fingernails, or they reach for something to eat.

WHAT DOES HUNGER FEEL LIKE?
WHAT DOES FULL FEEL LIKE?

In one of Roth's workshops, participants put one small piece of chocolate in their mouths and left it there for ten minutes, *really* tasting it. People found this a startling experience. Some of them had stuffed themselves with sweets. Many found that when they allowed themselves to eat something they wanted, slowly, actually enjoying it, they discovered it was easier to realize when they'd had enough and then to stop eating. If they ate secretly or very fast or while doing something else, like watching television, they were not even enjoying their food.

Many people, from gourmet chefs to research scientists, have noticed the same problem about Americans and their eating: many Americans have no idea when they're hungry and when they're full. In *I'm, Like, So Fat*, Dianne Neumark-Sztainer writes about it, too. Portions have been supersized since the 1970s, not just at fast food restaurants but also at the fancy place your family celebrates big events. As a result, people have gotten used to eating more and more at a time. According to one study Neumark-Sztainer mentions, most very small children will stop eating when they're full, but older children and adults will eat more if the portion in front of them is bigger.

When Brian Wansink, author of *Mindless Eating: Why We Eat More Than We Think*, asked people from Chicago, Illinois, how they knew it was time to stop eating a meal, most said it was over when their plate was empty or when their television show was over. When he asked people from Paris, France, they said they'd stop eating when they weren't hungry anymore. Although French people eat chocolate, pastries, and foods rich in fat, they pay attention to their food portions and to what their bodies tell them. Heavier people in America *and* France paid more attention to external clues than the feeling of fullness.

An organization called Body Positive suggests on its Web site that people learn again to pay attention to their body's signals. It created a scale that goes from 0 (weak with hunger) to 9, which comes *after* "painfully full." In between are stages of hunger and fullness. If you let yourself get too hungry, the organization says, then you're likely to eat anything. If you're hungry, then you are ready to eat but also ready to think about what you want. Then you experience the stages of fullness, tasting everything and paying attention to when you've had enough. Like Roth and

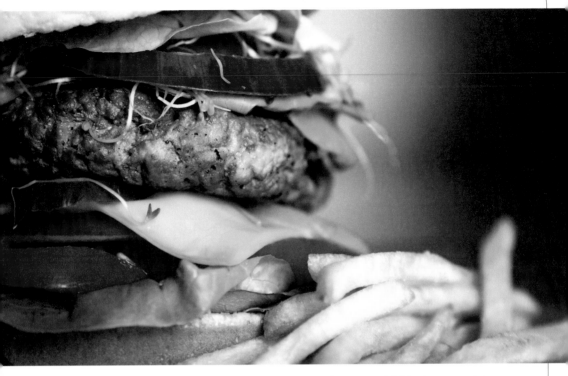

Does "eating well" mean you can never eat a cheeseburger again? No, but you might want to check the fat, sugar, and salt content of a fast-food burger/fries/soda meal and not eat one every day.

many others, the organization is suggesting that most Americans, especially people who have worried about their weight, don't really pay attention to what they eat. The popcorn you eat while watching a movie barely registers on your taste buds, but it registers on the scale.

WHEN YOU'RE NOT REALLY HUNGRY

So when you reach for a snack, what are you really doing? Are you really hungry? Can you pay attention and stop eating when you're full? If you're lonely or sad or worried or tired, then you

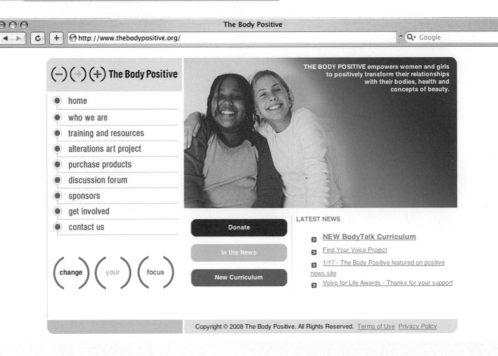

An organization called the Body Positive (www.thebodypositive.org) encourages people to feel better about their bodies, no matter what they weigh.

might find something that makes you feel better but that doesn't involve food. Call a friend. Pat the cat. Take a bath. Write in a journal. Watch a movie. Shoot hoops. Skate. Walk the dog. (Make your own list to be ready to combat the mindless munchies.)

Some of the things on the list involve physical activity. "You need exercise," everyone says. Exercise can be like dieting, though—something people do as though their body is an enemy they must conquer. Exercise doesn't have to be grim. It doesn't have to be something you stop as soon as you can. It's OK if you enjoy it.

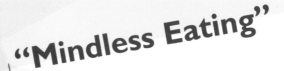

"Mindless Eating"

In 2006, a researcher named Brian Wansink published *Mindless Eating: Why We Eat More Than We Think*. In it, he tells of research experiments whose results he published in scientific journals. In one experiment, he gave people bowls of tomato soup that refilled (through a hose under the table) as they ate. People would eat until the experiment was over. They didn't feel fuller than the other participants, who had a normal bowl and had eaten a little more than a cup of soup. (One man did notice that the soup was rather filling, but he didn't know that he'd eaten more than a quart of it.) When Wansink had showed people the bowls, which held—or looked like they held—18 ounces (510 grams) and asked them how much they'd eat, most said they'd eat it all or they'd eat half of it. Only a few said they'd stop eating when they were full.

When you first learned to walk and then to run, you didn't do it because someone said it was good for you. Some young people keep that love of motion. And some had different amounts to start with. (Jean Mayer, a research scientist at Harvard, noted in the 1960s that some babies were thin but ate and moved a lot. Others were quieter and heavier and ate less.)

If you have lost your love of motion, you can try to find it again. Part of liking to move is habit. It's what you're used to. If you're not used to walking quickly or dancing or kickboxing, then when you start, you are going to be using muscles that you haven't been using. As you get into the habit of being more

47

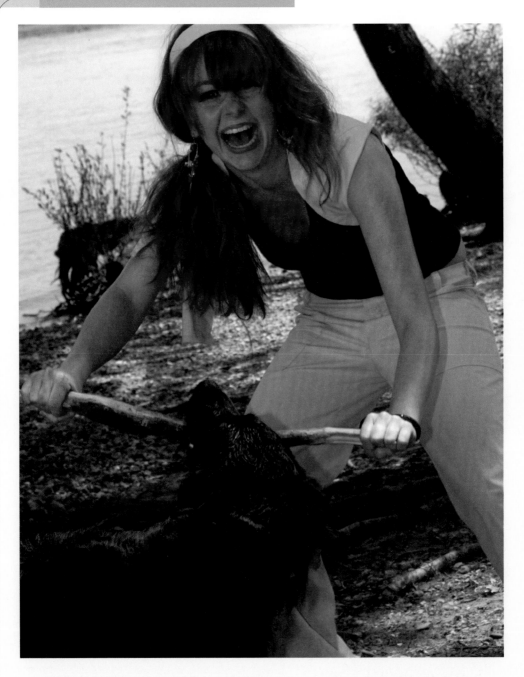

Being more active doesn't mean you have to exercise at the gym. Playing with your dog or a child you babysit for is good for you.

active, your body gets used to that. Many of the teens with whom Anne Fletcher talked said they missed being active if they were cooped up for a few days. Start slowly, she suggests. If you really haven't been getting exercise, you might be tired after five minutes of dancing or running. That's fine. When you can do it for a half hour, you'll have accomplished a lot. Be proud.

Physical activity makes your heart beat faster. It pumps blood and oxygen to your muscles and to your brain. Sometimes, when you're tired, you'll take a snack when you really need a nap. Other times, if you've been sitting too long in class or talking to friends, what you may need is to air your brain.

Researchers at the Mayo Clinic in Minnesota say regular exercise is helpful in many ways. Some of these are the following:

- It improves your mood. Exercise causes your brain to release chemicals that make you more relaxed and less stressed out.
- Exercise combats many of the diseases that the obesity researchers have associated with being overweight. These include controlling blood pressure and blood sugar. It also strengthens your bones, muscles, heart, and lungs.
- Exercise helps you sleep better.
- Exercise helps with weight management.

This last advantage to exercise can actually get people into trouble. You do burn more calories running than you do sitting, but walking (at 3.5 miles [5.6 kilometers] per hour) burns only about 280 calories, some of which you would have burned just sitting still (http://www.caloriesperhour.com). In other words, although exercise can indeed be part of weight management and is a part of good health, people tend to think that exercise is much more helpful for weight loss than it is. (According to Gary Taubes's article entitled "The Scientist and the Stairmaster" in *New York Magazine*, "the relationship between exercise and weight is 'more complex'" than many people suppose.) Sometimes, when people start getting more physical activity, they are discouraged when the exercise doesn't make them lose weight. If you start getting a lot of exercise, you will be burning some extra calories, but the other advantages are more important. Exercise will make you feel better. It can help you feel better about yourself and your body. It's fun to watch muscles develop. It's a good feeling when you go to pick up the bag of kitty litter or the gallon of milk and you think it must be empty because it seems too light. No, you're just stronger.

AN IMPROVED SELF-IMAGE

The message from Roth, Neumark-Sztainer, Fletcher, and many others is that people—adults, teens, children—will eat better and feel better if they can relearn how to feel hungry, how to enjoy what they eat, and how to know when they're full. That way, they will take pleasure in eating and they will also feel more in control of it. This isn't the kind of control that comes from eating with a fork in one hand and a calorie chart in the other. It isn't the kind of pleasure that you see on a television commercial that shows you how eating the newest magic product will change your life.

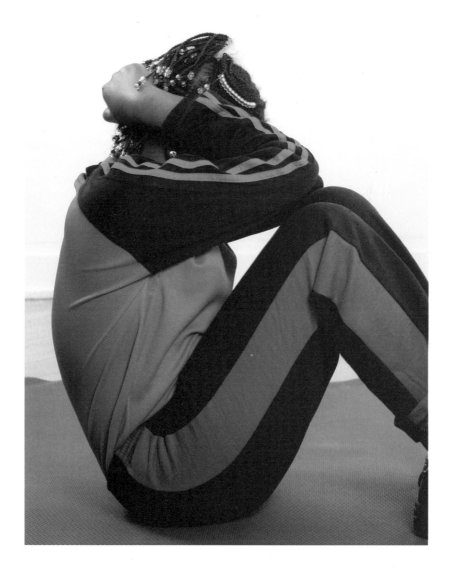

Some teens like to work out with weights and do other exercises to strengthen their muscles. "I feel strong" is a better statement for your self-image than "I feel fat."

The loudest voices from television and magazines make it easy to feel bad about yourself. They say: Consume more! Weigh less! Look perfect!

You can also choose to ignore these voices and can enjoy being your real self, in your real body, and enjoy taking care of it.

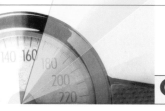

Glossary

binge To eat rapidly large amounts of food during a short period of time.

calories The units of energy that are released when the body breaks down food.

commitment To make a promise to do something.

confidential Private; told only to a limited number of people.

conform To act, dress, or think like others.

deprive To take away from; to deny.

diabetes An illness in which the body cannot process sugar and other carbohydrates. Type 1 diabetes usually develops in childhood, is caused by decreased insulin production, and is treated with insulin injections. Type 2 diabetes used to be found in older adults, but it is being seen more commonly in overweight adolescents and young adults. It is due to insulin resistance and can usually be managed by changes in eating habits.

discourage To take away hope; literally, to take away courage.

harass To bother constantly as by teasing, by making rude remarks, or by physically attacking.

irritable Grumpy; bad-tempered.

lifestyle A way of life that reflects someone's attitudes, beliefs, and identity.

media The plural of medium, which includes all the forms of mass communications, such as newspapers, radio, television, and magazines.

nutrition The process by which animals, including human beings, take in the food they need; the scientific study of what foods are needed.

obesity An excessive accumulation and storage of fat in the body.

perception Seeing; how what is seen is understood and interpreted.

perfect Totally without flaws; absolutely can't be improved.

stereotype An overly simple and often incorrect image.

yo-yo dieting A habit of losing weight by dieting, followed by regaining weight, and often repeating this pattern.

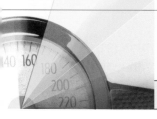

For More Information

About-Face
P.O. Box 77665
San Francisco, CA 94107
(415) 436-0212
Web site: http://www.about-face.org
About-Face promotes positive self-esteem in girls and women of all ages, sizes,
    races, and backgrounds through a spirited approach to media education,
    outreach, and activism.

The Alliance for Eating Disorders Awareness
P.O. Box 13155
North Palm Beach, FL 33408-3155
(866) 662-1235
Web site: http://www.eatingdisorderinfo.org
This organization tries to establish easily accessible programs in the United
    States that allow children and young adults the opportunity to learn
    about eating disorders and the positive effects of a healthy body image.
    Its aim is to disseminate educational information to the public about the
    warning signs, dangers, and consequences of anorexia, bulimia, and other
    related disorders, including exercise addiction.

Anorexia Nervosa and Related Eating Disorders, Inc. (ANRED)
P.O. Box 5102
Eugene, OR 97405
(541) 344-1144
Web site: http://www.anred.com

ANRED is a nonprofit organization, founded in 1979, that wants to make it easier for people to learn about eating disorders and how to recover from them. Officers include a psychiatrist, a clinical psychologist, a psychiatric nurse practitioner, a registered nurse who works in a mental health agency, and a pastoral counselor/eating disorders specialist.

Body Positive

P.O. Box 7801

Berkeley, CA 94707

(510) 528-0101

Web site: http://www.thebodypositive.org

Body Positive encourages teens to pursue "health at every size," by eating well, becoming physically active, and developing healthy self-respect and a positive body image.

Council on Size and Weight Discrimination

P.O. Box 305

Mt. Marion, NY 12456

(845) 679-1209

Web site: http://www.cswd.org

This nonprofit group works to change people's attitudes about weight.

National Association to Advance Fat Acceptance (NAAFA), Inc.

P.O. Box 22510

Oakland, CA 94609

(916) 558-6880

Web site: http://www.naafa.org

The NAAFA was founded in 1969 as a human rights organization dedicated to eliminating discrimination based on body size and to empowering people to accept themselves and promote acceptance of fat people within society.

**National Association of Anorexia Nervosa
and Associated Disorders (ANAD)**

P.O. Box 7

Highland Park, IL 60035

(847) 831-3438

Web site: http://www.anad.org

ANAD is the oldest eating disorder organization in the United States. Its president
and founder, Vivian Meehan, was a nurse at a hospital in Highland Park,
Illinois, when her daughter developed anorexia nervosa, and she discovered
there was no information available for sufferers or families. Today, ANAD
answers thousands of hotline calls each year and assists individuals and
their families to find resources and provide referrals to professionals.

National Eating Disorders Association (NEDA)

603 Stewart Street, Suite 803

Seattle, WA 98101

(800) 931-2237

Web site: http://www.nationaleatingdisorders.org

NEDA works to prevent eating disorders and provide treatment referrals to those
suffering from anorexia, bulimia, and binge eating disorder, and those
concerned with body image and weight issues. It is dedicated to expanding
public understanding and prevention of eating disorders and promoting
access to quality treatment for those affected, along with support for their
families through education, advocacy, and research.

Web Sites

Due to the changing nature of Internet links, Rosen Publishing
has developed an online list of Web sites related to the subject of
this book. This site is updated regularly. Please use this link to
access the list:

http://www.rosenlinks.com/uno/obsi

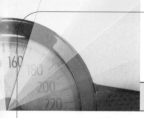

For Further Reading

Beck, Debra. *My Feet Aren't Ugly: A Girl's Guide to Loving Herself from the Inside Out.* New York, NY: Beaufort Books, 2007.

Boutaudou, Sylvie. *Weighing In: How to Understand Your Body, Lose Weight, and Live a Healthier Lifestyle.* New York, NY: Harry N. Abrams, 2006.

Crutcher, Chris. *Staying Fat for Sarah Byrnes.* New York, NY: HarperTeen, 2003.

Gay, Kathlyn. *Am I Fat? The Obesity Issue for Teens.* Berkeley Heights, NJ: Enslow, 2006.

Harmon, Daniel E. *Obesity* (Coping in a Changing World). New York, NY: Rosen Publishing, 2007.

Kirberger, Kimberly, ed. *No Body's Perfect: Stories by Teens About Body Image, Self-Acceptance, and the Search for Identity.* New York, NY: Scholastic, 2003.

Maloney, Michael, and Rachel Kranz. *Straight Talk About Eating Disorders.* New York, NY: Facts On File, 1991.

Nichter, Mimi. *Fat Talk: What Girls and Their Parents Say About Dieting.* Cambridge, MA: Harvard University Press, 2000.

Normandi, Carol, and Laurelee Roark. *Over It: A Teen's Guide to Getting Beyond Obsession with Food and Weight.* Novato, CA: New World Library, 2001.

Owens, Peter. *Teens: Health and Obesity.* Broomall, PA: Mason Crest, 2005.

Rutledge, Jill Zimmerman. *Picture Perfect: What You Need to Feel Better About Your Body.* Deerfield Beach, FL: HCI Health Communications, 2007.

Salmon, Margaret B. *Food Facts for Teenagers: A Guide to Good Nutrition for Teens and Preteens.* 2nd ed. Springfield, IL: Charles C. Thomas, 2003.

Schlosser, Eric, and Charles Wilson. *Chew on This.* New York, NY: Houghton Mifflin, 2006.

Tecco, Betsy Dru. *Food for Fuel: The Connection Between Food and Physical Activity.* New York, NY: Rosen Publishing, 2005.

Wansink, Brian. *Mindless Eating: Why We Eat More Than We Think.* Rev. ed. New York, NY: Bantam, 2007.

Youth Communication. *I Took Dieting Too Far* (Teens Write About Obesity and Self Image). New York, NY: Youth Communication/NY Center, 2005.

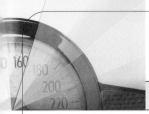

Bibliography

Allison, D. B., K. R. Fontaine, J. E. Manson, J. Stevens, T. B. VanItallie. "Annual Deaths Attributable to Obesity in the United States." *Journal of the American Medical Association*, Vol. 282, No. 16, 1999, pp. 1530–1538.

Campos, Paul. *The Obesity Myth*. New York, NY: Penguin, 2004.

Flegal, Katherine M., Barry I. Graubard, David F. Williamson, and Mitchell H. Gail. "Excess Deaths Associated with Underweight, Overweight, and Obesity." *Journal of the American Medical Association*, Vol. 293, 2005, pp. 1861–1867.

Fletcher, Anne M. *Weight Loss Confidential*. Boston, MA: Houghton Mifflin, 2006.

Gibbs, W. Wayt. "Obesity: An Overblown Epidemic?" *Scientific American*, May 23, 2005. Retrieved January 16, 2008 (http://www.sciam.com/article.cfm?articleID=000E5065-2345-128A-9E1583414B7F0000).

Harding, Anne. "Body Satisfaction Reflects Self-Esteem for Most Teens." Reuters.com, May 10, 2007. Retrieved December 2, 2007 (http://www.reuters.com/article/healthNews/idUSSPI05924420070510).

Kirschenbaum, Daniel S. "Do Overweight Children Have Lower Self-Esteem Than Non-Overweight Children?" Retrieved October 22, 2007 (http://www.myoverweightchild.com/self-esteem.html).

Kulick, Don, and Anne Meneley, eds. *Fat: The Anthropology of an Obsession*. New York, NY: Penguin, 2005.

Neumark-Sztainer, Dianne. *"I'm, Like, So Fat!" Helping Your Teen Make Healthy Choices About Eating and Exercise in a Weight-Obsessed World*. New York, NY: Guilford Press, 2005.

Phillips, Stone. "Who's to Blame for the U.S. Obesity Epidemic?" *Dateline*, August 19, 2006. Retrieved January 16, 2008 (http://www.msnbc.msn.com/id/14415766).

Pope, H. G., R. Olivardia, A. Gruber, and J. Borowiecki. "Evolving Ideals of Male Body as Seen Through Action Toys." *International Journal of Eating Disorders*, Vol. 26, 1999, pp. 65–72.

Powell, Lisa M., Glen Szczypka, Frank J. Chaloupka, and Carol L. Braunschweig. "Nutritional Content of Television Food Advertisements Seen by Children and Adolescents in the United States." *Pediatrics*, Vol. 120, Issue 3, September 2007, p. 576.

Roth, Geneen. "Make Peace with Your Body." Good Housekeeping. Retrieved January 2008 (http://www.goodhousekeeping.com/health/advice/feed-your-soul-0707).

Roth, Geneen. *When You Eat at the Refrigerator, Pull Up a Chair*. New York, NY: Hyperion, 1999.

Schwartz, Hillel. *Never Satisfied: A Cultural History of Diets, Fantasies, and Fat*. New York, NY: Doubleday, 1986.

Strauss, Richard S. "Childhood Obesity and Self-Esteem." *Pediatrics*, Vol. 105, No. 1, January 2000.

Taubes, Gary. "The Scientist and the Stairmaster." *New York Magazine*, September 24, 2007. Retrieved January 16, 2008 (http://nymag.com/news/sports/38001/index3.html).

Wansink, Brian. *Mindless Eating: Why We Eat More Than We Think*. Rev. ed. New York, NY: Bantam, 2007.

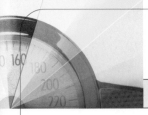

Index

About the Author

Judith Levin is a writer living in Brooklyn, New York. She has written numerous books for Rosen and other publishers, including *All You Need to Know About Diabetes*. While writing *Obesity and Self-Image*, she performed a three-month-long experiment: she never weighed herself, ate lots of fresh fruits and vegetables from farm stands, and ate all the cookies she wanted. At the end of three months, she was tired of cookies, craved fruits and vegetables, and hadn't changed her weight.

Photo Credits

Editor: Kathy Kuhtz Campbell; Photo Researcher: Marty Levick